The Cancer Wellness Cookbook

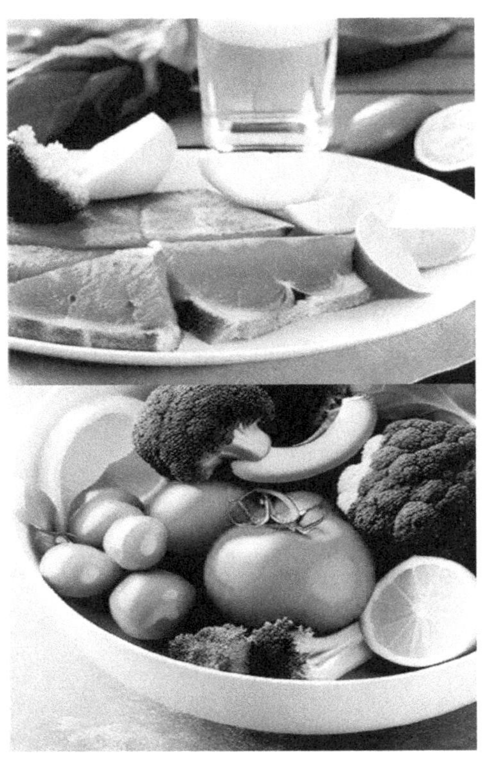

Smart Nutrition and Delicious Recipes for People Living with Cancer

Sham Billy

Table of Contents

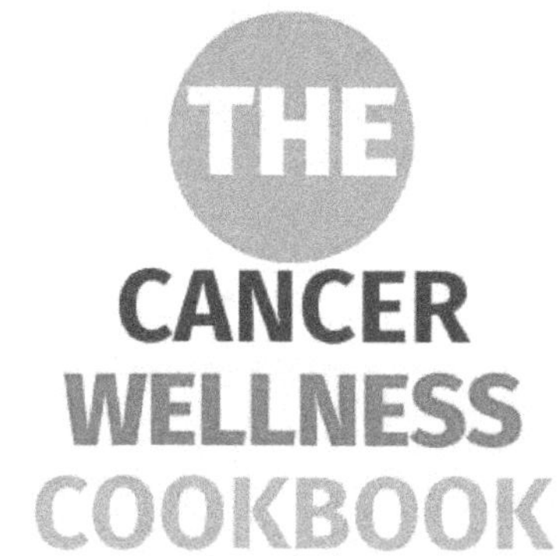
THE
CANCER
WELLNESS
COOKBOOK

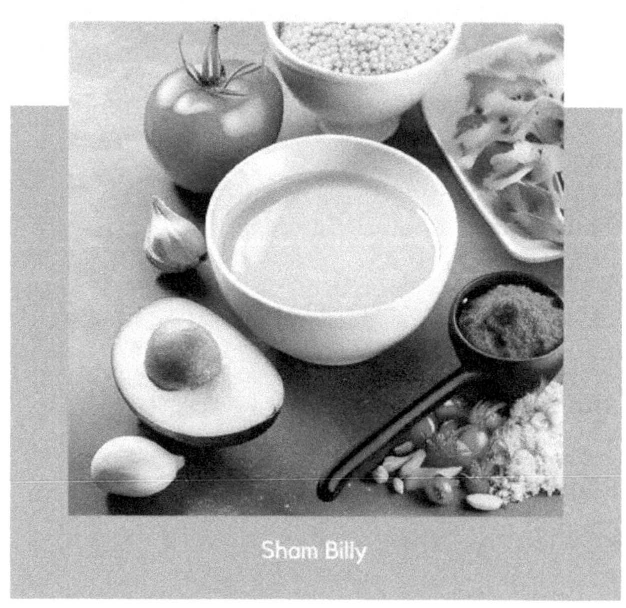
Sham Billy

Introduction

Ryan had been battling cancer for over a year. It was a tough journey, and he had gone through multiple rounds of chemotherapy and radiation. He had always been a foodie, but his cancer treatment had made it challenging to enjoy his favorite foods. He was constantly feeling tired and nauseous, and the thought of cooking a healthy meal seemed daunting.

One day, while browsing the internet, Ryan stumbled upon The Cancer Wellness Cookbook. He was intrigued by the title and decided to give it a try. He purchased the book and started to read through it immediately. The Cancer Wellness Cookbook was different from any other cookbook Ryan had ever seen. It was specifically designed to help cancer patients and survivors eat healthy and nourishing meals during and after cancer treatment. The recipes were not only delicious but also easy to make, with simple ingredients that were easy to find.

Ryan was excited to try out some of the recipes, and he started with the Tomato and Basil Soup. It was light, easy to digest, and had all the nutrients his body needed. As he continued to cook from the book, he noticed a significant improvement in his energy levels, and the nausea he had been experiencing started to fade away.

The Cancer Wellness Cookbook had become Ryan's go-to guide for healthy eating during and after his cancer treatment. He continued to experiment with new recipes and found that he was enjoying food once again. The book had helped him to understand the importance of eating a balanced diet and how it could help him to fight cancer.

Months passed, and Ryan's cancer went into remission. He was overjoyed, and he knew that The Cancer Wellness Cookbook had played a significant role in his recovery. He even recommended the book to his support group, and they all agreed that the recipes were not only tasty but also helped them to feel better during their treatment.

Ryan's journey with cancer had been tough, but with the help of The Cancer Wellness Cookbook, he had managed to overcome it. He was grateful for stumbling upon the book on the internet and for the nourishing meals it had helped him to create.

I. Introduction

Cancer is a complex disease that affects millions of people around the world. When someone is diagnosed with cancer, it can be overwhelming and confusing. In addition to medical treatments such as chemotherapy, radiation, and surgery, proper nutrition can play an important role in supporting the body's ability to fight cancer and promoting overall well-being. This is where "The Cancer Wellness Cookbook: Smart Nutrition and Delicious Recipes for People Living with Cancer" comes in.

About This Book:

"The Cancer Wellness Cookbook" is a comprehensive guide to smart nutrition and delicious recipes designed specifically for people living with cancer. This cookbook is written by Kimbrough Daniels, a certified oncology nutritionist and culinary expert, who has worked with cancer patients for over a decade. The book provides practical advice and easy-to-follow recipes to help support the nutritional needs of cancer patients and survivors.

The Cancer Wellness Cookbook is organized into 12 chapters, each focusing on a different aspect of cancer nutrition and wellness. These chapters cover everything from stocking your kitchen with essential ingredients and tools to meal planning and support resources. In addition, the book offers over 100 healthy and delicious recipes for breakfast, lunch, dinner, snacks, and beverages, all of which are designed to be easy to prepare and modify based on individual needs.

Understanding Cancer and Nutrition:

Cancer and its treatments can affect the body's ability to absorb and use nutrients, which can lead to malnutrition and a weakened immune system. Proper nutrition can help counteract these effects, promote healing, and improve quality of life. The Cancer Wellness Cookbook offers detailed information on cancer and nutrition, including the role of specific nutrients in the body, how cancer and its treatments can affect nutrition, and strategies for maintaining a healthy diet during and after treatment.

For example, the book explains how cancer and chemotherapy can cause nausea, vomiting, and taste changes, which can make it difficult to eat enough food. The book offers practical tips for managing these side effects, such as eating smaller, more frequent meals, avoiding strong smells and flavors, and experimenting with new foods and cooking methods. Additionally, the book emphasizes the importance of staying hydrated and offers suggestions for flavorful beverages that can help replenish fluids.

Tips for Using This Cookbook:

The Cancer Wellness Cookbook is designed to be a practical and user-friendly resource for people living with cancer. To help users get the most out of the book, it offers several tips and suggestions for using the recipes and information. For example, the book recommends reading through the entire recipe before beginning to cook, as well as organizing ingredients and tools in advance to make cooking easier.

The book also offers suggestions for modifying recipes to meet individual needs and preferences. For example, many of the recipes can be adapted for vegetarian or vegan diets, and the book provides tips for substituting ingredients based on dietary restrictions or allergies. Additionally, the book encourages readers to experiment with different flavors and ingredients, and to make adjustments based on personal taste.

How to Modify Recipes for Your Needs:

One of the key features of The Cancer Wellness Cookbook is its flexibility and adaptability. The book recognizes that everyone's nutritional needs and preferences are different, and offers suggestions for modifying recipes to meet individual needs. For example, the book suggests using low-sodium broth or reducing the amount of salt in recipes for people with high blood pressure or kidney problems. Additionally, the book provides guidance on modifying recipes to accommodate dietary restrictions or food allergies.

For example, if someone is lactose intolerant, the book suggests using dairy-free alternatives such as almond milk or soy milk in recipes that call for milk or cream. Similarly, if someone is allergic to nuts, the book offers suggestions for substituting seeds or other ingredients in recipes that contain nuts. The book also provides guidance on adjusting recipes for people who have difficulty swallowing or chewing, such as pureeing soups or blending smoothies.

In summary, "The Cancer Wellness Cookbook: Smart Nutrition and Delicious Recipes for People Living with Cancer" is a comprehensive resource for anyone looking to improve their nutrition and overall well-being while living with cancer. With its practical advice, easy-to-follow recipes, and suggestions for modifying recipes to meet individual needs, the book provides a wealth of information and inspiration for people looking to support their health through diet and lifestyle choices. By incorporating the tips and strategies outlined in this book, cancer patients and survivors can take an active role in their own health and well-being, and enjoy delicious, nourishing meals along the way.

II. The Cancer-Fighting Kitchen

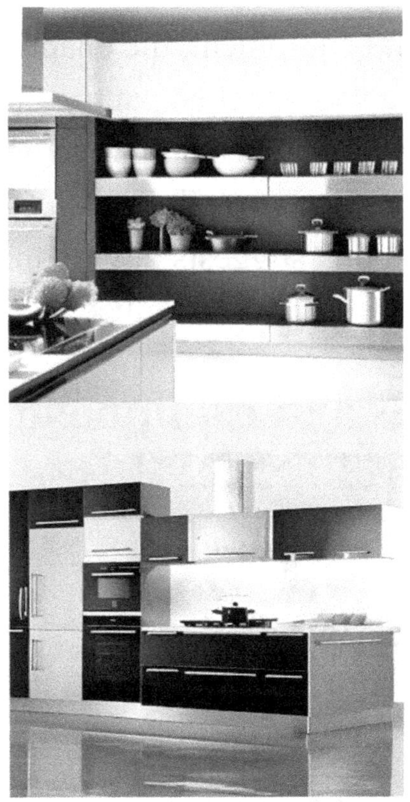

The kitchen is the heart of the home, and when it comes to cancer nutrition, it can also be a powerful tool for healing and wellness. In "The Cancer Wellness Cookbook," the chapter on the Cancer-Fighting Kitchen provides a comprehensive guide to stocking your kitchen with essential tools, ingredients, and flavor boosters that can help support your health and well-being during and after cancer treatment.

Stocking Your Kitchen:

The Cancer-Fighting Kitchen chapter begins by outlining the basic tools and equipment that are essential for any cancer patient or survivor's kitchen. These include items such as a good chef's knife, cutting board, vegetable peeler, and mixing bowls. The chapter also offers suggestions for other tools and appliances that can make cooking easier and more enjoyable, such as a blender, food processor, or immersion blender.

In addition to tools and equipment, the chapter emphasizes the importance of keeping a well-stocked pantry and refrigerator. This includes having a variety of canned and dried goods such as beans, lentils, whole grains, and nuts, as well as fresh fruits and vegetables, herbs, and spices. The book suggests buying in bulk and freezing extras to save money and reduce food waste.

Tools and Equipment:

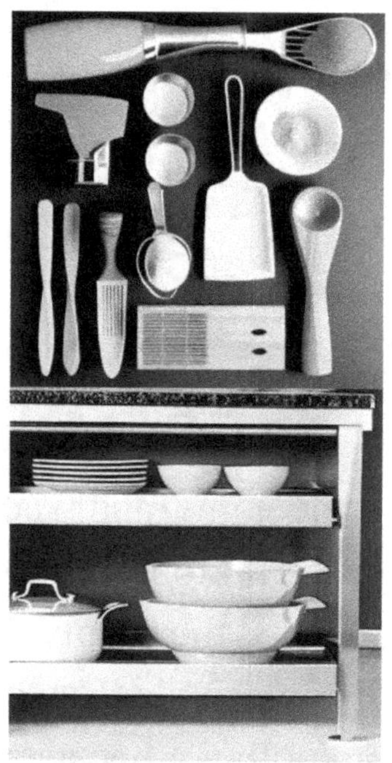

The Cancer-Fighting Kitchen chapter goes into further detail on the specific tools and equipment that can make cooking and meal preparation easier and more enjoyable for cancer patients and survivors. This includes items such as a garlic press or microplane grater for adding flavor to dishes, a vegetable steamer for retaining nutrients, and a slow cooker for making easy, healthy meals.

The chapter also emphasizes the importance of using non-toxic and non-reactive cookware and utensils, such as stainless steel, glass, or ceramic, to minimize exposure to harmful chemicals and substances. The book also provides tips for cleaning and storing kitchen tools and equipment to ensure food safety and longevity.

Essential Ingredients:

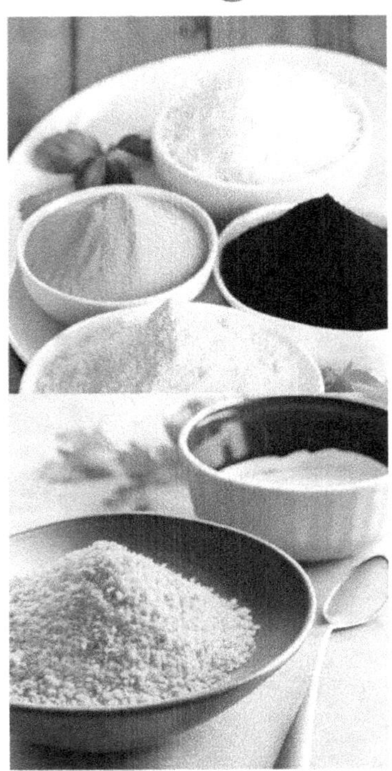

The Cancer-Fighting Kitchen chapter provides a detailed list of essential ingredients that are particularly beneficial for cancer patients and survivors. These include foods that are high in antioxidants, vitamins, minerals, and other nutrients that support the immune system, promote healing, and reduce inflammation. Some examples of these foods include:

1.   Leafy greens such as kale, spinach, and collard greens
2.   Cruciferous vegetables such as broccoli, cauliflower, and Brussels sprouts
3.   Berries such as blueberries, raspberries, and strawberries

4.   Whole grains such as quinoa, brown rice, and whole wheat pasta

5.   Legumes such as beans, lentils, and chickpeas

6.   Nuts and seeds such as almonds, walnuts, chia seeds, and flaxseeds

7.   Healthy fats such as avocado, olive oil, and coconut oil

The chapter also provides guidance on choosing high-quality, organic, and non-GMO ingredients whenever possible, as well as tips for buying and storing fresh produce to maximize freshness and nutrient content.

Flavor Boosters:

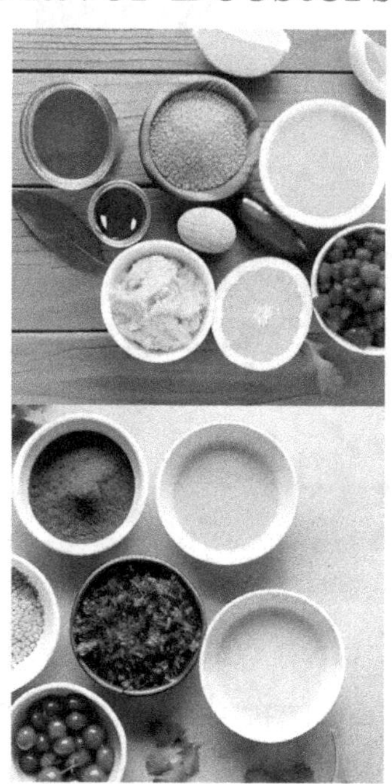

One of the challenges of cooking during and after cancer treatment is maintaining appetite and enjoyment of food, which can be affected by changes in taste, smell, and texture. The Cancer-Fighting Kitchen chapter offers a range of flavor boosters that can help enhance the taste and appeal of dishes, while also providing health benefits. These include ingredients such as:

1.   Citrus fruits such as lemons and limes, which can add brightness and acidity to dishes
2.   Vinegars such as apple cider or balsamic, which can add tang and depth of flavor
3.   Aromatics such as garlic, ginger, and onions, which can add complexity and depth of flavor
4.   Umami-rich ingredients such as miso, tamari, and nutritional yeast, which can add savory and meaty flavors
5.   Sweeteners such as honey, maple syrup, or dates, which can add sweetness without the use of refined sugars

The chapter also offers suggestions for using herbs and spices to add flavor and nutrition to dishes. For example, turmeric is a spice that has been shown to have anti-inflammatory properties, while cinnamon can help regulate blood sugar levels. Other herbs and spices that are particularly beneficial for cancer patients and survivors include basil, rosemary, thyme, and oregano.

Herbs and Spices:

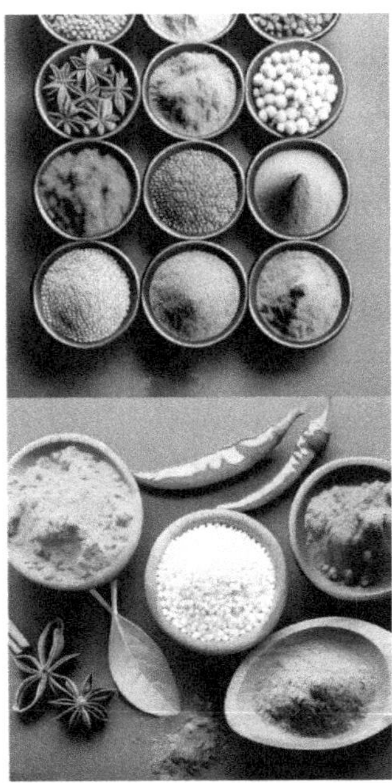

The Cancer-Fighting Kitchen chapter devotes a section to the health benefits of herbs and spices, which have been used for centuries for both culinary and medicinal purposes. The chapter provides a comprehensive list of herbs and spices that can be particularly beneficial for cancer patients and survivors, including:

Turmeric: This bright yellow spice has been shown to have anti-inflammatory properties, and may help reduce the risk of certain types of cancer.

Ginger: This root is well-known for its ability to soothe nausea and improve digestion, making it a great addition to meals for cancer patients undergoing chemotherapy or radiation.

Cinnamon: This spice has been shown to help regulate blood sugar levels, which can be particularly important for cancer patients who are at risk for developing type 2 diabetes.

Rosemary: This herb is rich in antioxidants, which can help protect against cellular damage and inflammation.

Thyme: This herb has antibacterial and anti-inflammatory properties, and may also help improve respiratory health.

Oregano: This herb is rich in antioxidants and has been shown to have antibacterial and anti-inflammatory properties.

Basil: This herb is rich in vitamin C and other antioxidants, and may also have anti-inflammatory properties.

In addition to their health benefits, herbs and spices can also add flavor and complexity to dishes without the use of added salt, sugar, or fat. The Cancer-Fighting Kitchen chapter provides tips for using herbs and spices in a variety of dishes, from soups and stews to salads and side dishes.

In summary, the Cancer-Fighting Kitchen chapter of "The Cancer Wellness Cookbook" provides a comprehensive guide to stocking your kitchen with essential tools, ingredients, and flavor boosters that can help support your health and well-being during and after cancer treatment. By focusing on nutrient-dense foods, non-toxic cookware, and a variety of flavor-enhancing ingredients, cancer patients and survivors can create meals that are both delicious and healing.

III. Breakfast and Brunch

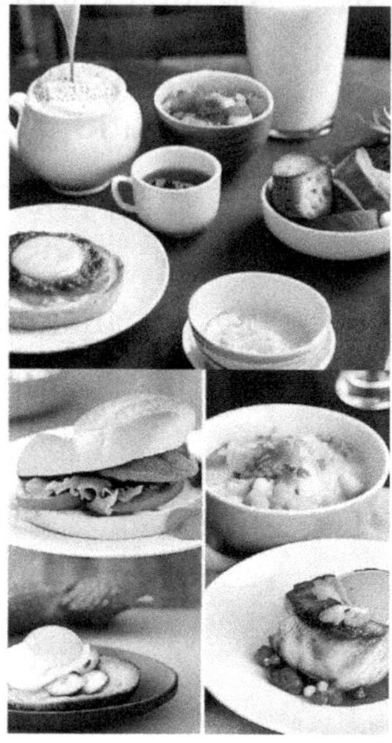

Breakfast is often referred to as the most important meal of the day, and it is especially important for cancer patients and survivors to start their day with a nutritious and satisfying meal. In "The Cancer Wellness Cookbook," the chapter on Breakfast and Brunch provides a variety of recipes and ideas for delicious and healthy breakfast options.

Smoothies and Juices:

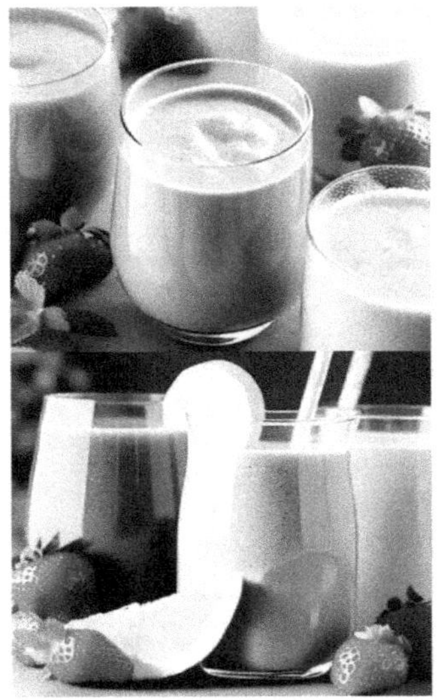

Smoothies and juices are a quick and easy way to start your day with a nutrient-dense and delicious meal. The Breakfast and Brunch chapter offers a variety of recipes for smoothies and juices that are packed with vitamins, minerals, and antioxidants. These recipes include ingredients such as leafy greens, fruits, nuts, and seeds.

One example of a cancer-fighting smoothie is the Berry Blast Smoothie, which includes blueberries, strawberries, almond milk, and chia seeds. This smoothie is high in antioxidants and fiber, which can help reduce inflammation and support digestive health.

Hot Breakfast Dishes:

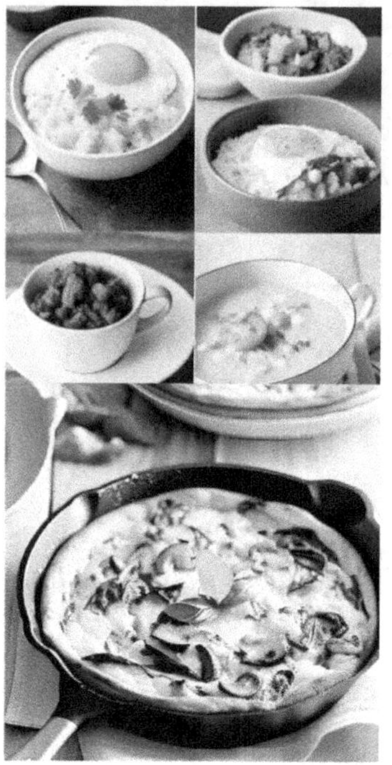

For those who prefer a hot breakfast, the Breakfast and Brunch chapter provides a variety of recipes for warming and comforting dishes. These dishes are often rich in protein and healthy fats, which can help maintain energy levels and support muscle recovery.

One example of a hot breakfast dish is the Mushroom and Spinach Frittata, which includes eggs, mushrooms, spinach, and Parmesan cheese. This dish is high in protein and fiber, which can help keep you feeling full and satisfied throughout the morning.

Breads and Pastries:

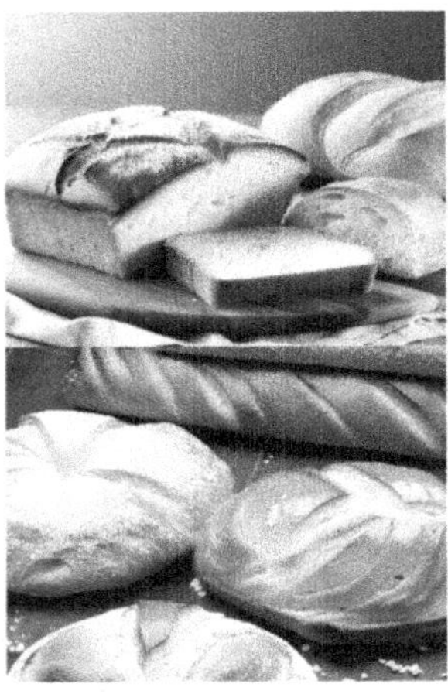

While many traditional breads and pastries can be high in sugar and refined carbohydrates, the Breakfast and Brunch chapter offers recipes for healthier and more nutritious options. These recipes use whole grains and natural sweeteners to provide sustained energy and fiber.

One example of a cancer-fighting bread is the Whole Wheat Banana Bread, which includes whole wheat flour, mashed bananas, and natural sweeteners such as honey or maple syrup. This bread is high in fiber and antioxidants, which can help support digestive health and reduce inflammation.

Brunch Favorites:

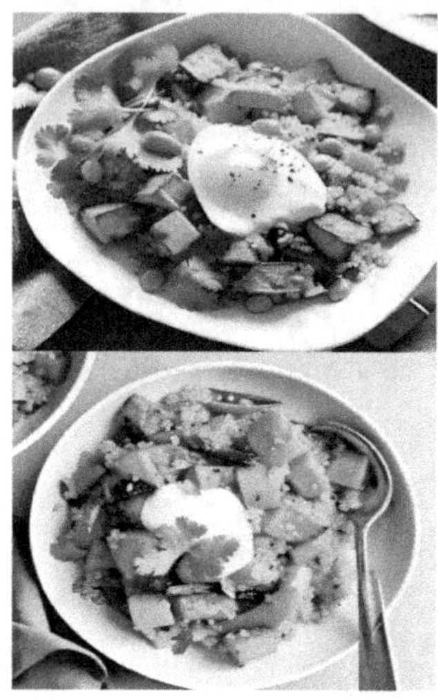

Brunch is a popular weekend tradition that often includes indulgent and decadent dishes. However, the Breakfast and Brunch chapter provides recipes for healthier and more nourishing brunch options that are still delicious and satisfying.

One example of a cancer-fighting brunch dish is the Quinoa and Sweet Potato Hash, which includes quinoa, sweet potatoes, onions, and spinach. This dish is high in fiber, protein, and vitamins, which can help support immune function and overall health.

Overall, the Breakfast and Brunch chapter provides a variety of recipes and ideas for healthy and delicious meals to start your day off on the right foot. Whether you prefer a smoothie, a hot breakfast dish, a healthy bread or pastry, or a nourishing brunch option, there is something for everyone in this chapter.

IV. Soups and Stews

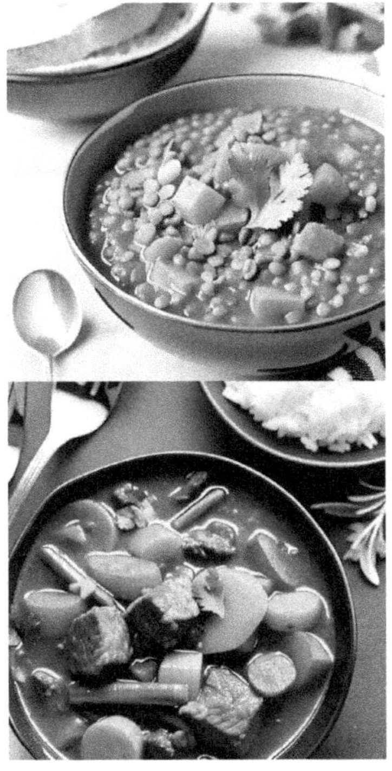

Soups and stews are some of the most comforting and nourishing dishes that can be enjoyed year-round. They are also an excellent way to incorporate a variety of nutritious ingredients into your diet, making them a great option for cancer patients and survivors. In this section, we will explore the different types of soups and stews that can be made to promote health and wellness.

Hearty and Nourishing Soups:

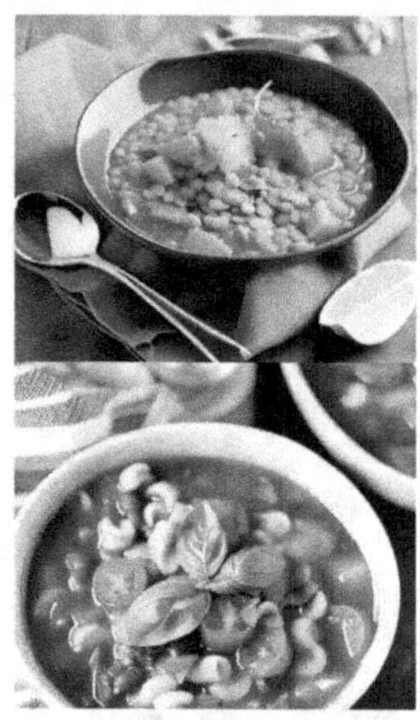

Hearty soups are perfect for colder months and provide warmth and comfort to the body. These soups typically include protein, complex carbohydrates, and healthy fats that can help keep you full and satisfied. Here are some examples of hearty soups that are perfect for cancer patients and survivors:

1. **Lentil Soup**: Lentils are an excellent source of plant-based protein and fiber, which can help support digestive health and reduce inflammation. Lentil soup can be made with a variety of vegetables and spices to add flavor and nutrients.

2. **Chicken Soup:** Chicken soup is a classic comfort food that is packed with nutrients. It can be made with homemade bone broth, which is rich in collagen, glucosamine, and other beneficial compounds that support gut health, joint health, and immune function.

3. **Minestrone Soup:** Minestrone soup is a hearty Italian soup that is packed with vegetables, beans, and whole grains. It is a great way to incorporate a variety of nutrient-dense foods into your diet and can be made with homemade vegetable broth for added health benefits.

Light and Refreshing Soups:

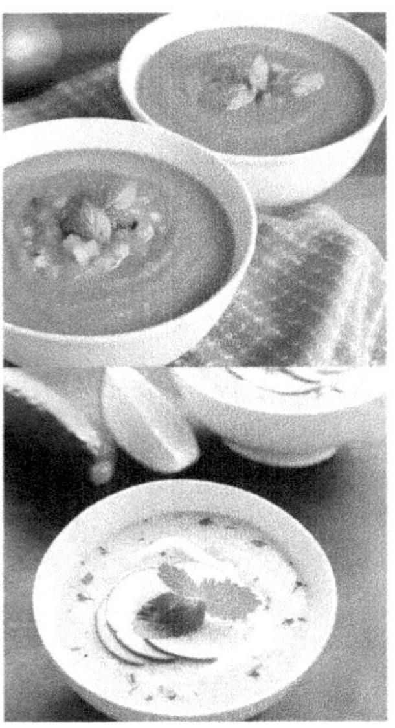

Light soups are perfect for warmer months when you want something refreshing and hydrating. These soups are typically made with vegetables and fruits that are high in water content and can help keep you cool and hydrated. Here are some examples of light soups that are perfect for cancer patients and survivors:

1.   **Gazpacho**: Gazpacho is a Spanish soup that is made with fresh vegetables such as tomatoes, cucumbers, and bell peppers. It is blended to a smooth consistency and served chilled, making it a refreshing and hydrating option for hot summer days.

2.   **Watermelon Soup**: Watermelon soup is a sweet and refreshing soup that is perfect for hot summer days. It is made with fresh watermelon, which is high in water content and packed with nutrients such as vitamin C, beta-carotene, and lycopene.

3.   **Cold Cucumber Soup:** Cold cucumber soup is a simple and refreshing soup that is made with fresh cucumbers, yogurt, and herbs. It is a great way to cool down on a hot day and provides a variety of health benefits such as hydration, gut health, and anti-inflammatory properties.

Stews and Chilis:

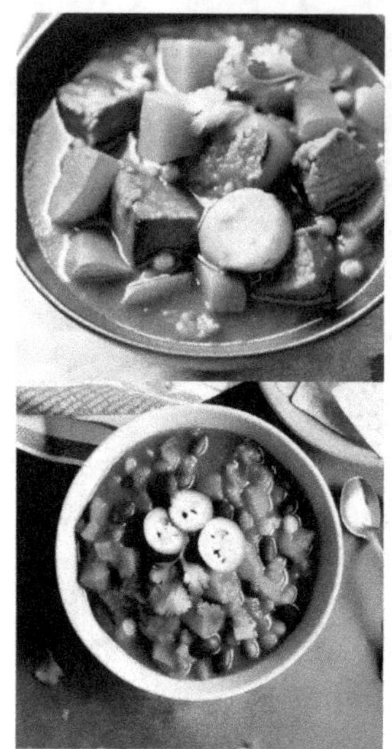

Stews and chilis are hearty dishes that are perfect for colder months and can be made with a variety of ingredients to provide a range of nutrients. They are typically made with a base of vegetables, beans or lentils, and meat or other protein sources. Here are some examples of stews and chilis that are perfect for cancer patients and survivors:

1.   **Beef Stew:** Beef stew is a classic comfort food that is packed with nutrients. It can be made with a variety of vegetables such as carrots, potatoes, and onions, and is typically simmered for several hours to develop rich flavors and tender meat.

2.   **Vegetarian Chili**: Vegetarian chili is a plant-based version of traditional chili that is made with a variety of beans and vegetables. It can be seasoned with a variety of spices such as cumin, chili powder, and paprika to add flavor and complexity.

3.   **Lentil Stew:** Lentil stew is a hearty and filling stew that is made with lentils and a variety of vegetables. It is an excellent source of plant-based protein and fiber, which can help support digestive health

and reduce inflammation. Lentil stew can also be made with a variety of spices and herbs to add flavor and nutrients.

Tips for Making Soups and Stews:

1.   Use homemade bone broth or vegetable broth for added health benefits and flavor.
2.   Incorporate a variety of colorful vegetables and fruits to provide a range of nutrients.
3.   Add spices and herbs such as turmeric, ginger, and garlic for added flavor and health benefits.
4.   Use lean protein sources such as chicken, fish, and beans for added nutrition and to keep the dish lighter.
5.   Don't be afraid to experiment with different ingredients and flavors to find your perfect soup or stew recipe.

In summary, soups and stews are a comforting and nourishing way to incorporate a variety of nutrient-dense foods into your diet. Whether you prefer a hearty and warming soup or a light and refreshing option, there are plenty of recipes to choose from that can support your health and wellness. By using a variety of colorful vegetables and fruits, lean protein sources, and spices and herbs, you can create delicious and nutritious soups and stews that are perfect for cancer patients and survivors.

V. Salads and Dressings

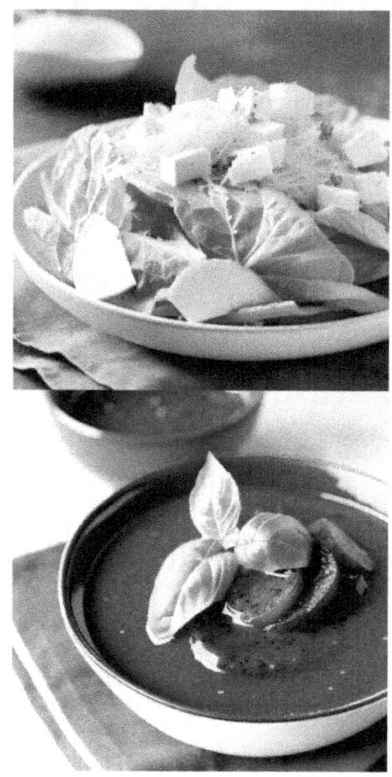

Salads are a great way to incorporate a variety of nutritious ingredients into your diet. They can be enjoyed as a main dish or as a side dish and can be customized to your preferences. Homemade dressings can also add flavor and nutrition to your salads. In this section, we will explore the different types of salads and dressings that can be made to promote health and wellness.

Classic Salads:

Classic salads are typically made with traditional ingredients and are a staple in many households. They are easy to make and can be enjoyed year-round. Here are some examples of classic salads that are perfect for cancer patients and survivors:

Caesar Salad: Caesar salad is a classic salad that is made with romaine lettuce, croutons, Parmesan cheese, and Caesar dressing. It is a great way to incorporate leafy greens into your diet and can be made with a homemade dressing for added nutrition.

Greek Salad: Greek salad is a popular Mediterranean dish that is made with tomatoes, cucumbers, red onions, feta cheese, and olives. It is typically dressed with a simple vinaigrette made with olive oil and red wine vinegar, making it a healthy and flavorful option.

Cobb Salad: Cobb salad is a hearty salad that is made with chopped lettuce, avocado, bacon, chicken, hard-boiled eggs, and blue cheese. It is a great way to incorporate a variety of proteins and healthy fats into your diet.

Creative Combinations:

Creative salads are perfect for those who want to mix up their routine and try something new. These salads typically incorporate a variety of ingredients and can be made with different textures and flavors. Here are some examples of creative salads that are perfect for cancer patients and survivors:

Roasted Vegetable Salad: Roasted vegetable salad is made with a variety of roasted vegetables such as sweet potatoes, Brussels sprouts, and beets. It is typically served over a bed of greens and can be dressed with a homemade vinaigrette for added nutrition.

Fruit Salad: Fruit salad is a refreshing and sweet salad that is made with a variety of seasonal fruits such as berries, melons, and grapes. It is a great way to incorporate a variety of vitamins and minerals into your diet and can be dressed with a yogurt or honey dressing for added sweetness.

Quinoa Salad: Quinoa salad is a protein-packed salad that is made with cooked quinoa, vegetables, and herbs. It can be customized with different vegetables and proteins such as grilled chicken or chickpeas for added nutrition.

Homemade Dressings:

Homemade dressings are a great way to add flavor and nutrition to your salads. They can be made with a variety of ingredients and can be customized to your preferences. Here are some examples of homemade dressings that are perfect for cancer patients and survivors:

Balsamic Vinaigrette: Balsamic vinaigrette is a simple and flavorful dressing that is made with balsamic vinegar, olive oil, Dijon mustard, and honey. It can be used on a variety of salads and can be stored in the fridge for up to a week.

Greek Yogurt Dressing: Greek yogurt dressing is a healthy and creamy dressing that is made with Greek yogurt, lemon juice, garlic, and herbs. It is a great way to add protein and probiotics to your salad and can be customized with different herbs and spices.

Lemon and Olive Oil Dressing: Lemon and olive oil dressing is a simple and refreshing dressing that is made with lemon juice, olive oil, and herbs. It is a great way to add flavor and healthy fats to your salad and can be used on a variety of greens and vegetables.

Incorporating salads and dressings into your diet is a great way to promote health and wellness. They can help you increase your intake of fruits, vegetables, proteins, and healthy fats, which can provide a variety of vitamins, minerals, and nutrients that can help support your body during cancer treatment and recovery. Here are some tips for incorporating salads and dressings into your diet:

1.   Experiment with different greens: There are many different types of greens that you can use for your salads, including kale, spinach, arugula, and romaine lettuce. Try mixing different types of greens together for added flavor and nutrition.

2.   Add a variety of toppings: Add a variety of toppings to your salads, including fruits, nuts, seeds, and proteins such as chicken, fish, or tofu. This can help make your salad more filling and provide additional nutrients.

3.   Make your own dressing: Homemade dressings are a healthier alternative to store-bought dressings, which can be high in sodium, sugar, and unhealthy fats. Experiment with different herbs, spices, and vinegars to create your own unique dressing.

4.   Plan ahead: Preparing your salads and dressings ahead of time can make it easier to incorporate them into your daily routine. Consider preparing a large batch of dressing and storing it in the fridge for easy access throughout the week.

5.   Pair your salad with a healthy protein: Pairing your salad with a healthy protein source can help make it more filling and provide additional nutrients. Consider adding grilled chicken, salmon, or chickpeas to your salad for added protein.

In summary, salads and dressings are a delicious and nutritious way to incorporate a variety of ingredients into your diet. With a little creativity and experimentation, you can create your own unique salads and dressings that are perfect for cancer patients and survivors. By incorporating salads and dressings into your daily routine, you can help support your body during cancer treatment and recovery and promote long-term health and wellness.

VI. Vegetables and Sides

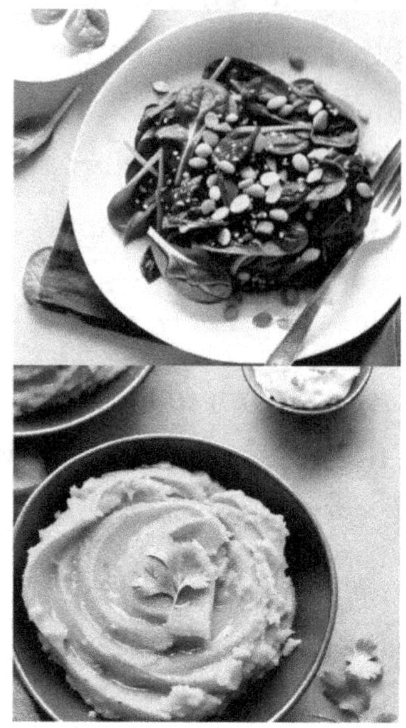

Vegetables and sides are an essential part of any healthy and balanced diet. They provide essential nutrients, fiber, and vitamins that are vital for overall health and wellbeing. In this section, we will explore some delicious and nutritious vegetables and side dishes that are perfect for cancer patients and survivors.

Roasted Vegetables:

Roasting vegetables is a simple and easy way to add flavor and nutrition to your diet. Roasting brings out the natural sweetness of vegetables and gives them a delicious caramelized flavor. Here are some examples of roasted vegetables that are perfect for cancer patients and survivors:

Roasted Broccoli: Broccoli is a cruciferous vegetable that is packed with cancer-fighting compounds. Roasting broccoli with garlic and olive oil is a simple and delicious way to enjoy this nutrient-dense vegetable.

Roasted Carrots: Carrots are an excellent source of beta-carotene, which is a potent antioxidant that helps to protect against cancer. Roasting carrots with honey and thyme is a tasty and nutritious side dish.

Roasted Brussel Sprouts: Brussel sprouts are a cruciferous vegetable that is rich in vitamin C and fiber. Roasting Brussel sprouts with balsamic vinegar and maple syrup is a sweet and savory dish that is perfect for fall.

Grilled and Sauteed Vegetables:

Grilling and sautéing vegetables is another simple and delicious way to add flavor and nutrition to your diet. Grilling adds a smoky flavor to vegetables, while sautéing helps to retain their natural flavors and nutrients. Here are some examples of grilled and sautéed vegetables that are perfect for cancer patients and survivors:

Grilled Asparagus: Asparagus is a nutrient-dense vegetable that is rich in antioxidants and fiber. Grilling asparagus with olive oil and lemon juice is a simple and tasty way to enjoy this healthy vegetable.

Sautéed Spinach: Spinach is a leafy green vegetable that is rich in iron, vitamin C, and antioxidants. Sautéing spinach with garlic and olive oil is a delicious and healthy side dish that can be enjoyed with any meal.

Grilled Portobello Mushrooms: Portobello mushrooms are a rich source of vitamins and minerals and are a great source of plant-based protein. Grilling portobello mushrooms with balsamic vinegar and herbs is a tasty and nutritious dish that can be enjoyed as a side or as a vegetarian main course.

Hearty Whole Grains:

Whole grains are an important part of a healthy and balanced diet. They are a great source of fiber, protein, and essential vitamins and minerals. Here are some examples of hearty whole grains that are perfect for cancer patients and survivors:

Quinoa: Quinoa is a gluten-free grain that is high in protein and fiber. It is also a good source of iron, magnesium, and calcium. Quinoa can be served as a side dish or used as a base for salads or bowls.

Brown Rice: Brown rice is a whole grain that is rich in fiber and essential nutrients. It is also a good source of antioxidants and can help to reduce the risk of cancer. Brown rice can be used as a base for stir-fries or as a side dish.

Barley: Barley is a hearty whole grain that is high in fiber and protein. It is also a good source of vitamins and minerals, including iron, magnesium, and selenium. Barley can be used in soups or stews or served as a side dish.

Comforting Starchy Sides:

Starchy sides are a comforting and satisfying addition to any meal. They provide energy and essential nutrients that are important for overall health and wellbeing. Here are some examples of comforting starchy sides that are perfect for cancer patients and survivors:

Mashed Sweet Potatoes: Sweet potatoes are a rich source of beta-carotene, which is a potent antioxidant that can help to protect against cancer. Mashing sweet potatoes with a touch of cinnamon and nutmeg is a tasty and nutritious side dish.

Roasted Potatoes: Potatoes are a good source of fiber, potassium, and vitamin C. Roasting potatoes with herbs and olive oil is a simple and delicious side dish that can be enjoyed with any meal.

Butternut Squash: Butternut squash is a rich source of vitamins A and C and is also high in fiber. Roasting butternut squash with brown sugar and cinnamon is a sweet and savory side dish that is perfect for fall.

In summary, vegetables and sides are an essential part of any healthy and balanced diet, especially for cancer patients and survivors. Roasting, grilling, and sautéing vegetables can bring out their natural flavors and add variety to your meals. Whole grains provide essential nutrients and fiber, while starchy sides are a comforting addition to any meal. By incorporating these nutritious and delicious options into your diet, you can help to support your overall health and wellbeing.

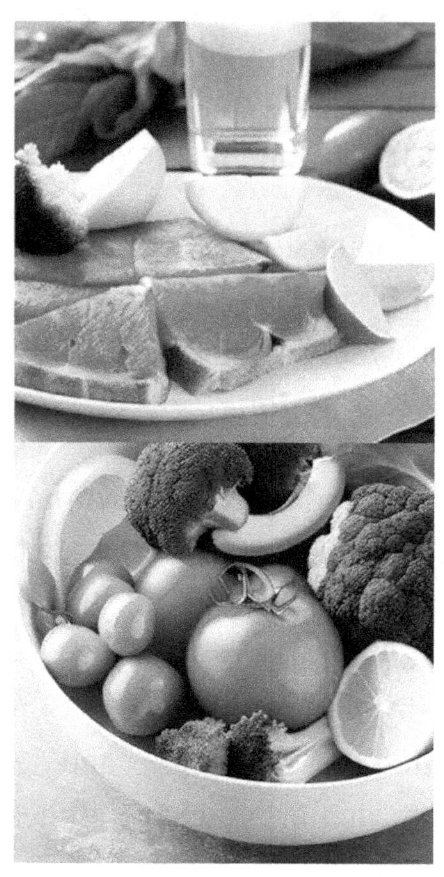

VII. Main Dishes

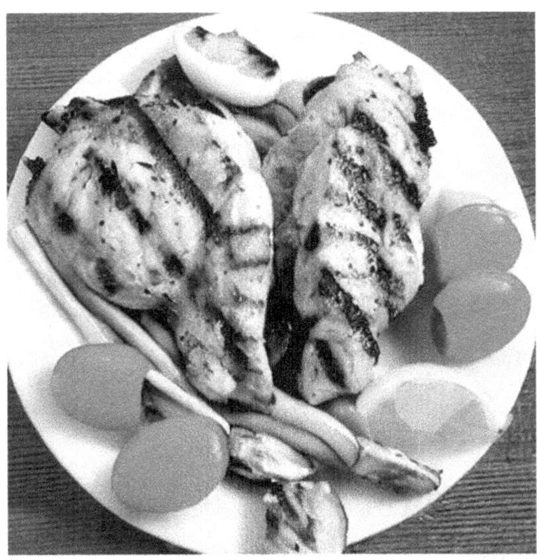

Main dishes are the centerpiece of any meal. They are often the most satisfying and filling part of a meal and provide a range of essential nutrients. In this section, we will explore some delicious and nutritious main dishes that are perfect for cancer patients and survivors.

Poultry and Meat:

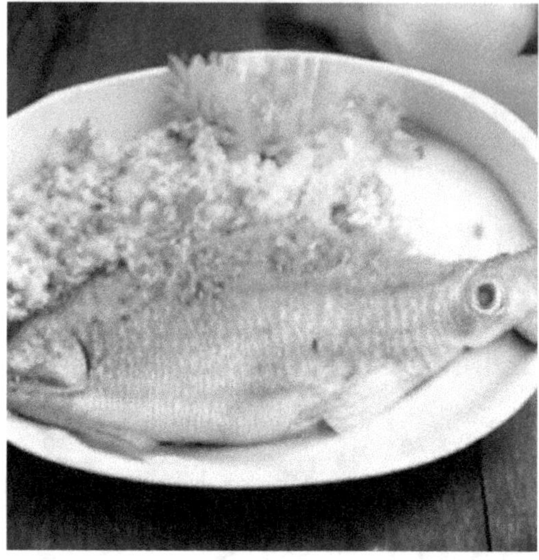

Poultry and meat are excellent sources of protein, which is essential for building and repairing tissues in the body. However, it is important to choose lean cuts of meat and poultry and avoid processed meats, which are high in sodium and saturated fat. Here are some examples of healthy and delicious poultry and meat dishes that are perfect for cancer patients and survivors:

Grilled Chicken: Grilled chicken is a healthy and delicious way to enjoy poultry. Chicken breast is a lean cut of meat that is high in protein and low in saturated fat. Grilled chicken can be marinated in a range of herbs and spices for added flavor.

Baked Fish: Fish is a good source of omega-3 fatty acids, which have been shown to reduce inflammation and lower the risk of cancer. Baked fish, such as salmon, cod, or tilapia, can be seasoned with herbs and lemon juice for a simple and healthy meal.

Lean Beef Stir-Fry: Lean beef is a good source of protein and iron. Stir-frying beef with a variety of vegetables, such as bell peppers, onions, and broccoli, is a tasty and nutritious way to enjoy this protein-rich food.

Seafood:

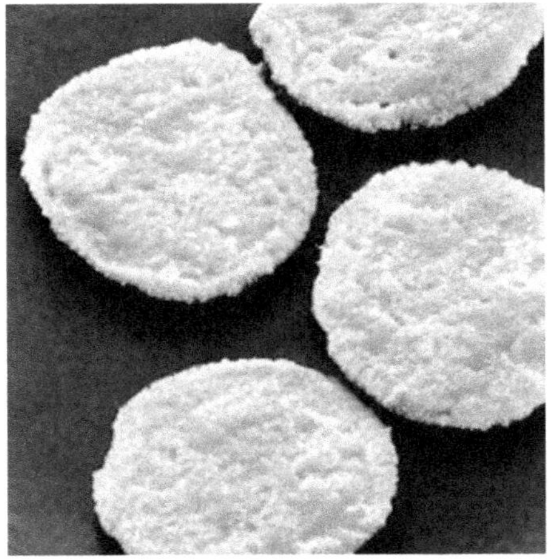

Seafood is a great source of protein, omega-3 fatty acids, and other essential nutrients. Seafood is also low in saturated fat and can help to reduce inflammation in the body. Here are some examples of healthy and delicious seafood dishes that are perfect for cancer patients and survivors:

Grilled Shrimp Skewers: Shrimp is a low-calorie and high-protein seafood that is easy to prepare. Grilled shrimp skewers can be marinated in a range of herbs and spices for added flavor.

Baked Cod: Cod is a lean white fish that is rich in protein and low in fat. Baked cod can be seasoned with herbs and lemon juice for a simple and healthy meal.

Salmon Patties: Salmon is a fatty fish that is rich in omega-3 fatty acids. Salmon patties can be made with canned salmon, which is an affordable and convenient option. These patties can be served with a side salad or whole-grain bun.

Vegetarian and Vegan:

A plant-based diet can provide a range of essential nutrients, including protein, fiber, and vitamins. Vegetarian and vegan dishes are also generally lower in saturated fat and can help to reduce inflammation in the body. Here are some examples of healthy and delicious vegetarian and vegan dishes that are perfect for cancer patients and survivors:

Roasted Vegetable Quinoa Bowl: Quinoa is a high-protein grain that is gluten-free and easy to digest. Roasted vegetables, such as sweet potatoes, Brussels sprouts, and cauliflower, can be added to a quinoa bowl for a filling and nutritious meal.

Vegetable Stir-Fry: Stir-frying vegetables, such as bell peppers, onions, and mushrooms, with a variety of herbs and spices is a tasty and healthy vegetarian option.

Vegan Chili: Chili can be made with a range of vegetables, such as tomatoes, bell peppers, onions, and beans, for a filling and nutritious meal. Vegan chili can be seasoned with a range of spices and served with a side of brown rice or quinoa.

Pasta and Noodles:

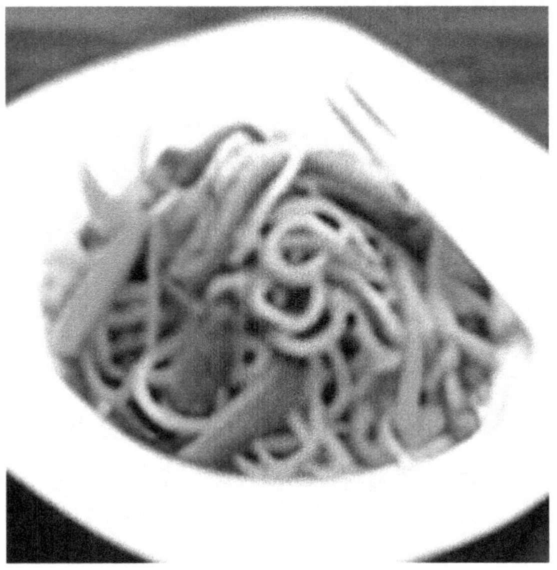

Pasta and noodles are a staple food in many cultures and can provide a range of essential nutrients, including carbohydrates and fiber. However, it is important to choose whole-grain pasta and avoid pasta dishes that are high in saturated fat and sodium. Here are some examples of pasta and noodle dishes that are perfect for cancer patients and survivors:

Whole Wheat Pasta with Tomato Sauce: Whole wheat pasta is a good source of fiber and can help to reduce the risk of cancer. Tomato sauce is rich in lycopene, which is a powerful antioxidant that can help to protect against cancer. To make this dish, cook whole wheat pasta according to package instructions and serve with homemade tomato sauce, made with fresh tomatoes, garlic, and olive oil.

Veggie Noodle Stir-Fry: Veggie noodle stir-fry is a tasty and nutritious dish that can be made with a variety of vegetables, such as broccoli, carrots, bell peppers, and mushrooms. Use whole-grain noodles or spiralized vegetables, such as zucchini or sweet potato, instead of traditional noodles. Add protein by including tofu, edamame, or nuts, and season with ginger, garlic, and soy sauce.

Pesto Pasta with Roasted Vegetables: Pesto is a delicious and flavorful sauce made with basil, garlic, and olive oil. To make this dish, roast a selection of vegetables, such as broccoli, bell peppers, and cherry tomatoes, and serve with whole-grain pasta and a homemade pesto sauce. Pesto is a good source of healthy fats, and the vegetables provide a range of essential nutrients.

Spaghetti Squash with Marinara Sauce: Spaghetti squash is a healthy and low-carb alternative to traditional pasta. To make this dish, cut a spaghetti squash in half, remove the seeds, and bake in the oven until tender. Use a fork to scrape the flesh into spaghetti-like strands, and serve with homemade marinara sauce made with fresh tomatoes, garlic, and herbs.

In summary, a healthy and balanced diet is essential for cancer patients and survivors. Including a variety of nutrient-dense foods, such as fruits, vegetables, whole grains, lean protein, and healthy fats, can help to reduce the risk of cancer, support the immune system, and improve overall health and wellbeing. By incorporating the examples of main dishes discussed in this article, cancer patients and survivors can enjoy delicious and nutritious meals that are packed with essential nutrients and flavor. As always, it is important to consult with a healthcare professional or a registered dietitian before making any major changes to your diet.

VIII. Snacks and Appetizers

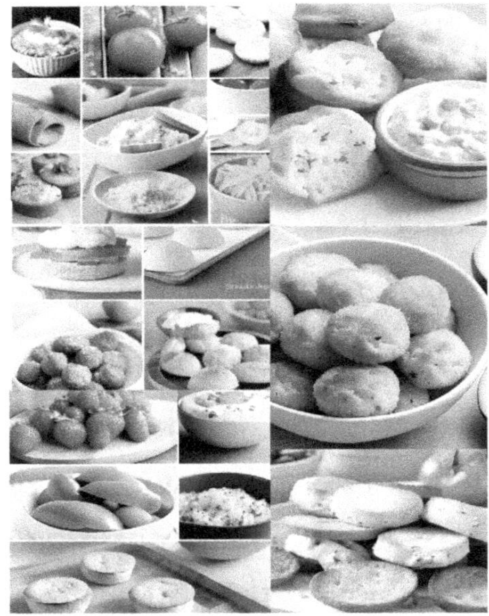

Snacks and appetizers are a great way to satisfy hunger and provide a quick energy boost between meals. However, it is important to choose healthy options that are rich in nutrients and avoid snacks that are high in sugar, salt, and saturated fat. In this section, we will explore some delicious and nutritious snacks and appetizers that are perfect for cancer patients and survivors.

Dips and Spreads:

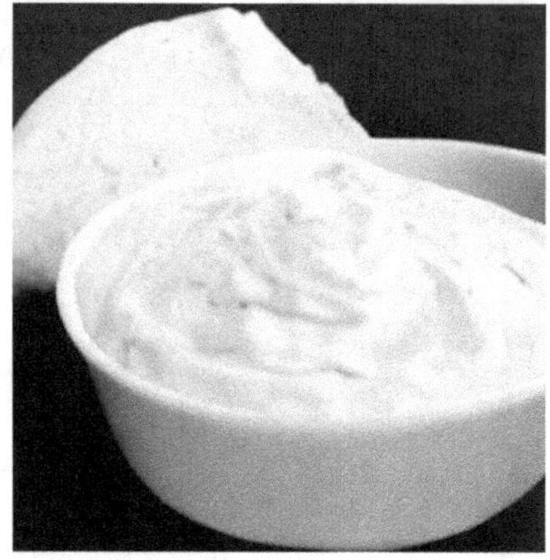

Dips and spreads are a versatile and delicious way to enjoy a range of healthy ingredients. They can be served with a variety of vegetables, crackers, and bread for a satisfying and nutritious snack. Here are some examples of dips and spreads that are perfect for cancer patients and survivors:

Hummus: Hummus is a Middle Eastern dip that is made from chickpeas, tahini, lemon juice, and garlic. It is high in protein, fiber, and healthy fats, and can be enjoyed with pita bread, crackers, or vegetables.

Guacamole: Guacamole is a Mexican dip that is made from avocados, lime juice, and spices. Avocados are high in healthy fats and fiber, and can help to reduce inflammation and improve heart health. Guacamole can be enjoyed with tortilla chips or vegetables.

White Bean Dip: White bean dip is a creamy and flavorful dip that is made from white beans, garlic, lemon juice, and herbs. White beans are high in protein, fiber, and antioxidants, and can help to lower cholesterol levels. White bean dip can be enjoyed with vegetables or crackers.

Savory Bites:

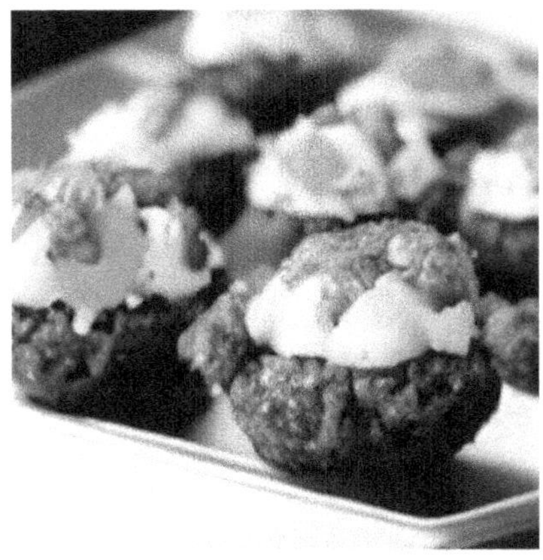

Savory bites are a delicious and satisfying way to enjoy a range of healthy ingredients. They can be made from a variety of ingredients, including vegetables, cheese, and whole grains. Here are some examples of savory bites that are perfect for cancer patients and survivors:

Stuffed Mushrooms: Stuffed mushrooms are a delicious and nutritious appetizer that can be made with a variety of fillings, including spinach, cheese, and herbs. Mushrooms are rich in vitamins and minerals, and can help to boost immunity and reduce inflammation.

Sweet Potato Bites: Sweet potato bites are a tasty and nutritious snack that can be made with roasted sweet potato slices and a variety of toppings, including cheese, herbs, and nuts. Sweet potatoes are high in fiber, vitamins, and antioxidants, and can help to regulate blood sugar levels.

Cucumber Bites: Cucumber bites are a refreshing and low-calorie snack that can be made with cucumber slices and a variety of toppings, including cream cheese, smoked salmon, and herbs. Cucumbers are high in water, fiber, and antioxidants, and can help to reduce inflammation and improve digestion.

Sweet Treats:

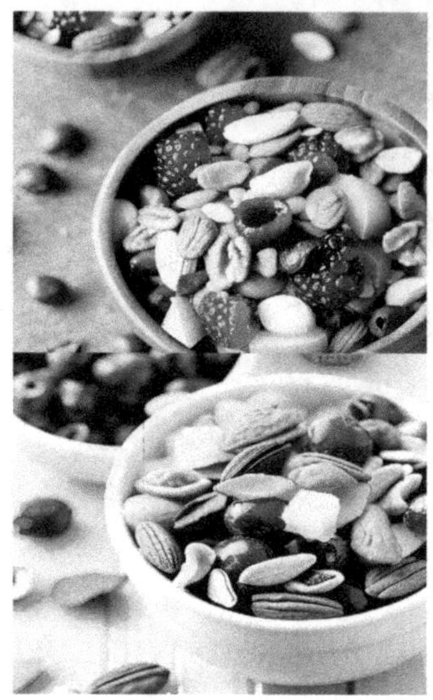

Sweet treats are a delicious way to indulge in a little bit of sweetness without compromising on nutrition. They can be made from a variety of ingredients, including fruits, nuts, and whole grains. Here are some examples of sweet treats that are perfect for cancer patients and survivors:

Fruit Salad: Fruit salad is a refreshing and nutritious dessert that can be made with a variety of fruits, including berries, melons, and citrus. Fruits are high in vitamins, minerals, and antioxidants, and can help to reduce inflammation and improve heart health.

Dark Chocolate: Dark chocolate is a delicious and nutritious treat that is high in antioxidants and can help to reduce inflammation and improve heart health. It is important to choose dark chocolate that is at least 70% cocoa and avoid varieties that are high in sugar and saturated fat.

Trail Mix: Trail mix is a tasty and nutritious snack that can be made with a variety of ingredients, including nuts, seeds, and dried fruits. Nuts are high in healthy fats, fiber, and protein, and can help to reduce inflammation and lower the risk of heart disease. Dried fruits provide natural sweetness and are a good source of fiber and vitamins. Seeds like pumpkin or sunflower seeds provide essential minerals like magnesium and zinc. Making your own trail mix is a great way to control the ingredients and make it suitable for your taste preferences and dietary restrictions.

To make a simple trail mix, start with a base of unsalted nuts such as almonds, walnuts, or cashews. Add in some dried fruits like raisins, cranberries, or apricots, and some seeds such as pumpkin or sunflower seeds. You can also add in some dark chocolate chips or coconut flakes for a sweet twist. Mix everything together and portion it out into individual snack bags for easy grab-and-go snacks.

Hummus and Veggies: Hummus is a tasty and nutritious dip that is made from chickpeas, tahini, lemon juice, and olive oil. It is a good source of protein, fiber, and healthy fats, and can be enjoyed with a variety of vegetables for a satisfying and nutritious snack.

To make homemade hummus, combine chickpeas, tahini, lemon juice, garlic, and olive oil in a food processor and blend until smooth. You can add in additional ingredients like roasted red peppers, roasted garlic, or herbs to add extra flavor. Serve with a variety of fresh vegetables like carrots, celery, cucumbers, or bell peppers for a healthy and satisfying snack.

Sweet Potato Fries: Sweet potato fries are a delicious and healthy alternative to traditional French fries. Sweet potatoes are a good source of fiber, vitamins, and antioxidants, and can help to regulate blood sugar levels.

To make sweet potato fries, cut sweet potatoes into thin strips and toss them in a bowl with a drizzle of olive oil and some seasonings like paprika or garlic powder. Spread the fries out in a single layer on a baking sheet and bake in the oven at 425°F for about 20-25 minutes, flipping halfway through. Serve with a dipping sauce like Greek yogurt ranch or honey mustard for a tasty and nutritious snack.

Bruschetta: Bruschetta is a classic Italian appetizer that is made with grilled bread and a tomato and basil topping. It is a simple and delicious snack that is perfect for entertaining or as a light meal.

To make bruschetta, slice a baguette into thin rounds and brush each slice with olive oil. Grill or toast the bread until lightly browned and crispy. In a bowl, mix diced tomatoes, fresh basil, garlic, olive oil, and balsamic vinegar. Spoon the tomato mixture onto the toasted bread and serve immediately for a delicious and satisfying snack.

Energy Balls: Energy balls are a healthy and convenient snack that is made from a mixture of nuts, seeds, and dried fruits. They are easy to make and can be customized with your favorite ingredients.

To make energy balls, start with a base of nuts and seeds such as almonds, cashews, chia seeds, or flaxseeds. Add in some dried fruits like dates or raisins for natural sweetness, and some flavorings like cocoa powder, coconut flakes, or vanilla extract. Pulse everything together in a food processor until it forms a sticky dough. Roll the mixture into bite-sized balls and store them in the fridge for a quick and nutritious snack on-the-go.

In summary, there are many healthy and tasty snack and appetizer options that can provide essential nutrients and energy for cancer patients and survivors. Choosing whole foods and avoiding processed and high-sugar snacks can help to promote overall health and wellbeing. Experiment with different ingredients and flavors to find your favorite snacks that you can enjoy guilt-free.

IX. Beverages:

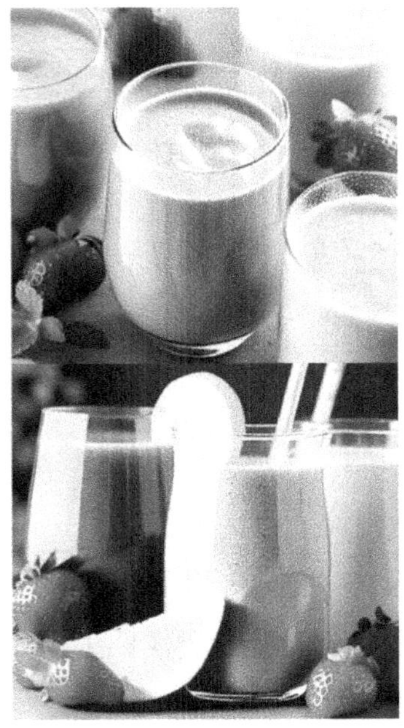

Beverages are an essential part of our daily diet and play a vital role in keeping us hydrated and healthy. Choosing the right beverages can provide us with essential nutrients and vitamins, while also being a source of pleasure and enjoyment. In this section, we will explore some delicious and nutritious beverage options that are perfect for cancer patients and survivors.

Infused Waters and Teas:

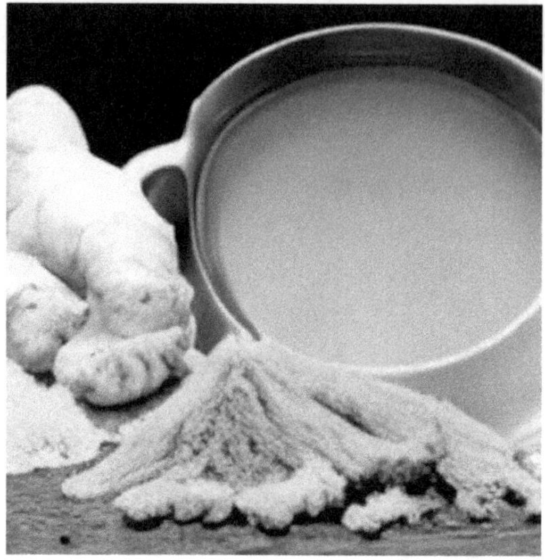

Infused waters and teas are a great way to stay hydrated while also enjoying the natural flavors and health benefits of fruits and herbs. Infused waters are easy to make and can be customized to your personal preferences. Here are some examples of infused waters and teas that are perfect for cancer patients and survivors:

Lemon and Mint Infused Water: Lemon and mint are both rich in antioxidants and can help to reduce inflammation in the body. Infusing water with lemon and mint is a refreshing and delicious way to stay hydrated.

Ginger and Turmeric Tea: Ginger and turmeric are both known for their anti-inflammatory and antioxidant properties. Brewing tea with fresh ginger and turmeric is a soothing and comforting beverage that can also help to reduce nausea and improve digestion.

Berry and Hibiscus Infused Water: Berries are rich in antioxidants and can help to reduce the risk of cancer. Hibiscus tea is also rich in antioxidants and can help to lower blood pressure. Infusing water with berries and hibiscus is a flavorful and nutritious way to stay hydrated.

Smoothies and Shakes:

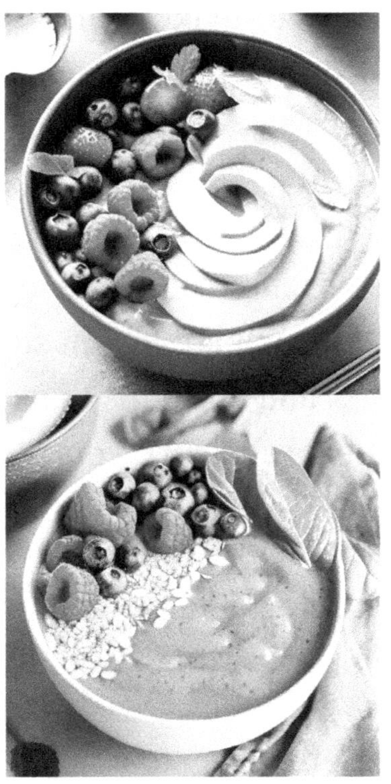

Smoothies and shakes are a delicious and nutritious way to get a variety of essential nutrients in one easy-to-make drink. Smoothies and shakes can be made with a variety of fruits, vegetables, and protein sources to meet your specific dietary needs. Here are some examples of smoothies and shakes that are perfect for cancer patients and survivors:

Green Smoothie: Green smoothies are a great way to get a variety of nutrients from leafy greens and fruits. Blend together spinach, kale, banana, and almond milk for a nutritious and delicious smoothie.

Berry Smoothie: Berries are rich in antioxidants and can help to reduce inflammation in the body. Blend together frozen berries, almond milk, and Greek yogurt for a healthy and satisfying smoothie.

Protein Shake: Protein shakes are a great way to get protein and essential nutrients in one easy-to-make drink. Blend together protein powder, almond milk, and frozen fruit for a quick and nutritious shake.

Juices and Cocktails:

Juices and cocktails can be a source of pleasure and enjoyment, but it is important to choose options that are low in sugar and alcohol. Here are some examples of juices and cocktails that are perfect for cancer patients and survivors:

Green Juice: Green juices are a great way to get a variety of nutrients from vegetables and fruits. Juicing kale, cucumber, apple, and lemon together can provide a nutritious and delicious juice.

Mocktail: Mocktails are a great way to enjoy a cocktail without the alcohol. Combine sparkling water, cranberry juice, and lime for a refreshing and low-sugar mocktail.

Herbal Cocktail: Herbal cocktails can provide a variety of health benefits from the herbs used. Muddle fresh herbs like basil or mint with fresh lime juice and soda water for a refreshing and healthy cocktail.

In summary, choosing the right beverages can be a simple and delicious way to stay hydrated and get essential nutrients in your diet. Infused waters and teas, smoothies and shakes, and juices and cocktails can all provide a variety of health benefits and can be customized to your personal preferences. When choosing your beverages, aim for options that are low in sugar and alcohol and choose ingredients that are rich in antioxidants and other essential nutrients.

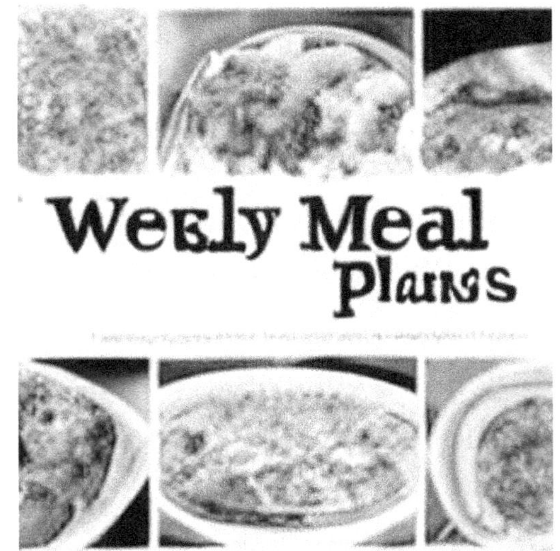

Meal planning is an important aspect of maintaining a healthy and balanced diet. Planning out your meals can help you save time, money, and reduce food waste. It also ensures that you have healthy and nutritious meals on hand, making it easier to stick to your dietary goals. In this section, we will explore various aspects of meal planning, including weekly meal plans, sample menus, shopping lists, and tips for successful meal planning.

Weekly Meal Plans:

Creating a weekly meal plan can be an effective way to stay on track with your dietary goals. A weekly meal plan allows you to plan out your meals for the week, making it easier to grocery shop and prepare your meals in advance. Here are some steps to follow when creating a weekly meal plan:

1.   **Decide on your dietary goals:** Before creating a meal plan, it is important to decide on your dietary goals. This could include goals

such as reducing your intake of processed foods, increasing your vegetable intake, or reducing your overall calorie intake.

2. **Plan your meals:** Once you have determined your dietary goals, you can begin planning your meals for the week. Choose a variety of foods from each food group, including vegetables, fruits, whole grains, lean proteins, and healthy fats.

3. **Write down your plan:** Write down your meal plan for the week, including breakfast, lunch, dinner, and snacks. Be sure to include any recipes or cooking instructions.

4. **Shop for groceries:** Once you have your meal plan, create a grocery list and shop for the ingredients you need.

5. **Prepare in advance**: To save time during the week, you can prepare some of your meals in advance, such as chopping vegetables or cooking grains.

Sample Menus:

Creating a sample menu can be a helpful way to plan out your meals for the week. A sample menu can also help you to stay on track with your dietary goals. Here are some examples of sample menus:

1. Sample Menu for Weight Loss:

Breakfast: Greek yogurt with berries and almonds

Snack: Carrot sticks with hummus

Lunch: Grilled chicken salad with mixed greens, tomatoes, and cucumbers

Snack: Apple slices with almond butter

Dinner: Grilled salmon with roasted vegetables and quinoa

2.   Sample Menu for Vegetarian Diet:

Breakfast: Oatmeal with sliced banana and almond milk

Snack: Trail mix with almonds, walnuts, and dried cranberries

Lunch: Lentil soup with whole-grain bread

Snack: Roasted chickpeas

Dinner: Tofu stir-fry with mixed vegetables and brown rice

Shopping Lists:

Creating a shopping list can help you to stay organized and ensure that you have all the ingredients you need for your meals. Here are some tips for creating a shopping list:

1.   **Plan your meals:** Before creating your shopping list, plan out your meals for the week. This will help you to determine what ingredients you need.
2.   **Check your pantry:** Before heading to the grocery store, check your pantry to see what ingredients you already have on hand.
3.   **Organize your list:** Organize your list by food group to make it easier to navigate the grocery store.
4.   **Stick to your list:** When at the grocery store, stick to your list to avoid impulse purchases.
5.   **Buy in bulk:** Consider buying ingredients in bulk, such as grains or nuts, to save money.

Tips for Meal Planning:

Here are some additional tips to help you with your meal planning:

1.   **Cook in batches:** Consider cooking in batches and freezing extra portions for later meals. This can save time and help you to avoid unhealthy takeout meals.

2.   **Use leftovers:** Use leftover ingredients to create new meals, such as using leftover chicken in a salad.

3.   **Keep it simple:** Focus on simple and easy-to-prepare meals. You don't have to make complicated recipes every day to eat well.

4.   **Plan for snacks:** Don't forget to plan for healthy snacks between meals. This can help to keep you satisfied and prevent overeating.

5.   **Use seasonal produce:** Take advantage of seasonal produce, which tends to be fresher, more flavorful, and less expensive.

6.   **Experiment with new recipes:** Try new recipes and ingredients to keep things interesting and prevent boredom with your meals.

7.   **Stay flexible**: Remember that your meal plan is a guide, not a strict rule. Stay flexible and make adjustments as needed based on your preferences and schedule.

8.   **Don't forget about hydration:** Along with meal planning, it's important to also plan for hydration. Aim to drink plenty of water throughout the day, and consider incorporating hydrating beverages such as infused waters and herbal teas into your meal plan.

9.   **Listen to your body:** Lastly, listen to your body and pay attention to how certain foods make you feel. Adjust your meal plan as needed to meet your individual needs and preferences.

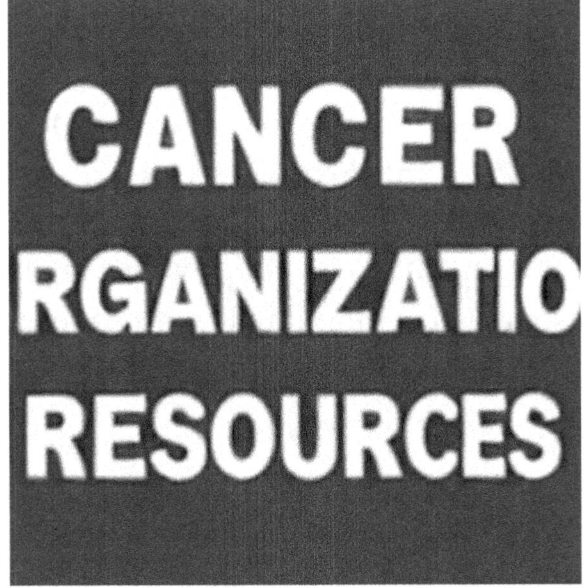

Cancer can be a challenging experience for both the person diagnosed and their loved ones. Proper nutrition and wellness resources can help to support individuals with cancer in their recovery journey. Additionally, support and community resources can help to reduce the feelings of isolation and provide a sense of belonging. In this section, we will explore some of the resources and support available to individuals with cancer.

Cancer Organizations and Resources:

There are many organizations and resources available to individuals with cancer. These organizations provide valuable information, resources, and support to help individuals navigate their cancer journey. Some of the most well-known cancer organizations include the American Cancer Society (ACS), National Cancer Institute (NCI), and CancerCare.

The American Cancer Society (ACS) is a nationwide organization dedicated to cancer research, education, and support. They offer a variety of resources for individuals with cancer, including information on treatment options, support groups, and financial assistance programs. The ACS also has a 24-hour helpline where individuals can speak with trained cancer information specialists for support and information.

The National Cancer Institute (NCI) is another organization that provides valuable resources for individuals with cancer. The NCI is the federal government's principal agency for cancer research and offers a range of resources on cancer prevention, screening, diagnosis, and treatment. The NCI also sponsors clinical trials for cancer treatment and provides information on how to participate.

CancerCare is a national non-profit organization that provides free professional support services to individuals with cancer, including counseling, financial assistance, and support groups. They offer support to individuals and their loved ones in coping with the emotional and practical challenges of a cancer diagnosis.

Nutrition and Wellness Resources:

Proper nutrition is essential for individuals with cancer as it can help to support the body's natural healing process and reduce the risk of infection. There are many nutrition and wellness resources available to individuals with cancer, including registered dietitians, cancer-specific nutrition programs, and alternative therapies.

Registered dietitians (RDs) are trained professionals who specialize in nutrition and can help individuals with cancer develop a healthy and balanced diet. RDs can also provide guidance on managing common side effects of cancer treatment, such as nausea and loss of appetite.

Cancer-specific nutrition programs, such as the Cancer Nutrition Consortium, offer resources and education on nutrition for individuals with cancer. These programs often provide customized nutrition plans and support for individuals undergoing cancer treatment.

Alternative therapies, such as acupuncture and massage, can also be beneficial for individuals with cancer. These therapies can help to reduce stress and anxiety, alleviate pain, and improve overall well-being.

Support and Community:

Support and community resources can be invaluable for individuals with cancer. These resources can provide emotional support, help to reduce feelings of isolation, and provide a sense of belonging. Some of the most common support and community resources include cancer support groups, online communities, and peer-to-peer support.

Cancer support groups are a valuable resource for individuals with cancer. These groups provide a safe and supportive environment for individuals to share their experiences and connect with others who are going through similar experiences. Many cancer organizations, such as the American Cancer Society and CancerCare, offer support groups for individuals with cancer and their loved ones.

Online communities, such as Cancer Survivors Network and MyLifeLine, provide a platform for individuals with cancer to connect with others and share their experiences. These communities can provide a sense of community and belonging, even for those who may be unable to attend in-person support groups.

Peer-to-peer support programs, such as the American Cancer Society's Reach to Recovery program, connect individuals with trained volunteers who have been through a similar cancer experience. These programs can provide emotional support, practical advice, and hope to individuals with cancer.

In summary, Navigating a cancer diagnosis can be a challenging experience, but there are many resources and support available to individuals and their loved ones. Nutrition is an important aspect of cancer care and can play a significant role in managing side effects and improving overall health and wellbeing.

There are various cancer organizations and resources that can provide information and guidance on nutrition and cancer care. These organizations also offer support groups and counseling services for patients and their families.

In addition to cancer-specific resources, there are also numerous nutrition and wellness resources available to help individuals make healthy choices and maintain a balanced diet. These resources can provide guidance on healthy eating habits, recipe ideas, and meal planning strategies.

Finally, support and community are critical components of cancer care. Finding a supportive network of friends, family, and healthcare professionals can provide emotional support and encouragement throughout the cancer journey.

Overall, the resources and support available for individuals with cancer can help to improve their quality of life and provide a sense of community during a difficult time. By taking a proactive approach to nutrition and seeking out support, individuals can better manage their cancer treatment and maintain their health and wellbeing.

XII. Conclusion

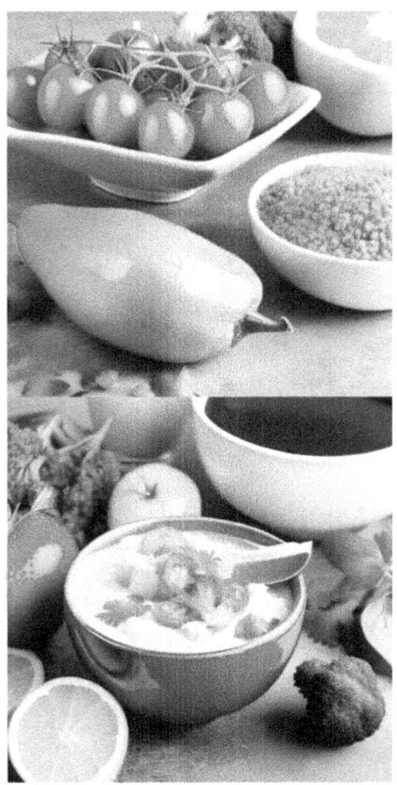

Final Thoughts:

Living with cancer can be a difficult journey, but it is important to remember that good nutrition can play a vital role in managing symptoms and supporting overall health. By incorporating a variety of healthy foods into your diet and working with a healthcare professional, you can optimize your nutrition and support your body's healing process.

Remember, healthy eating doesn't have to be complicated or expensive. With a little planning and preparation, you can create delicious and nutritious meals that will help you to feel your best.

Acknowledgments:

We would like to acknowledge the healthcare professionals, researchers, and individuals affected by cancer who have contributed to the development of this resource. Your dedication to improving the lives of those affected by cancer is greatly appreciated.

Recipe Index:

1. Grilled Salmon with Mango Salsa
2. Spinach and Feta Stuffed Chicken Breast
3. Quinoa and Black Bean Salad
4. Roasted Vegetable and Hummus Wrap
5. Turkey and Avocado Sandwich
6. Lentil Soup with Vegetables
7. Berry and Yogurt Parfait
8. Trail Mix
9. Infused Water with Lemon and Mint
10. Green Smoothie
11. Orange Carrot Juice
12. Strawberry Margarita

Glossary:

1. **Antioxidants**: Compounds that protect cells from damage caused by harmful molecules called free radicals.
2. **Carbohydrates**: A macronutrient that provides energy to the body.

3.   **Fiber**: A type of carbohydrate that is not digested by the body and helps to promote bowel regularity.

4.   **Macronutrients**: Nutrients that the body needs in large amounts, including carbohydrates, protein, and fat.

5.   **Micronutrients**: Nutrients that the body needs in smaller amounts, including vitamins and minerals.

6.   **Phytochemicals**: Compounds found in plant-based foods that may have health benefits.

7.   **Protein**: A macronutrient that is important for building and repairing tissues in the body.

8.   **Whole grains**: Grains that contain the entire grain kernel, including the bran, germ, and endosperm.

About the Author:

Sham Billy, MS, RD, is a registered dietitian with 8 years of experience in oncology nutrition. He has worked with individuals affected by cancer in various settings, including hospitals, cancer centers, and private practice. He is passionate about empowering individuals to make informed nutrition choices that support their health and well-being. In his free time, Sham Billy enjoys hiking, cooking, and spending time with her family.

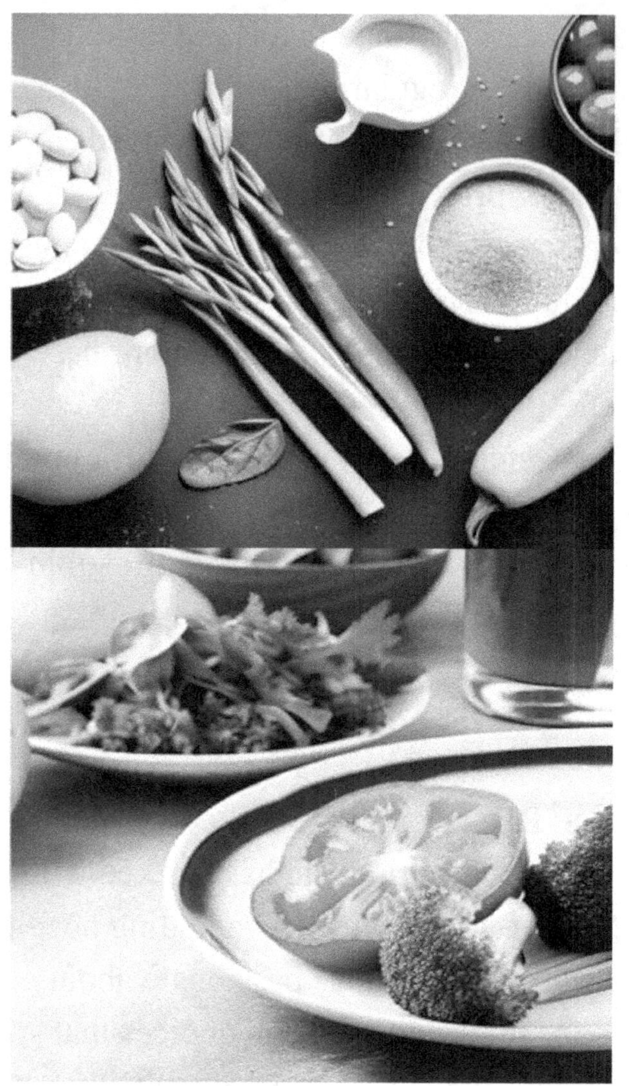

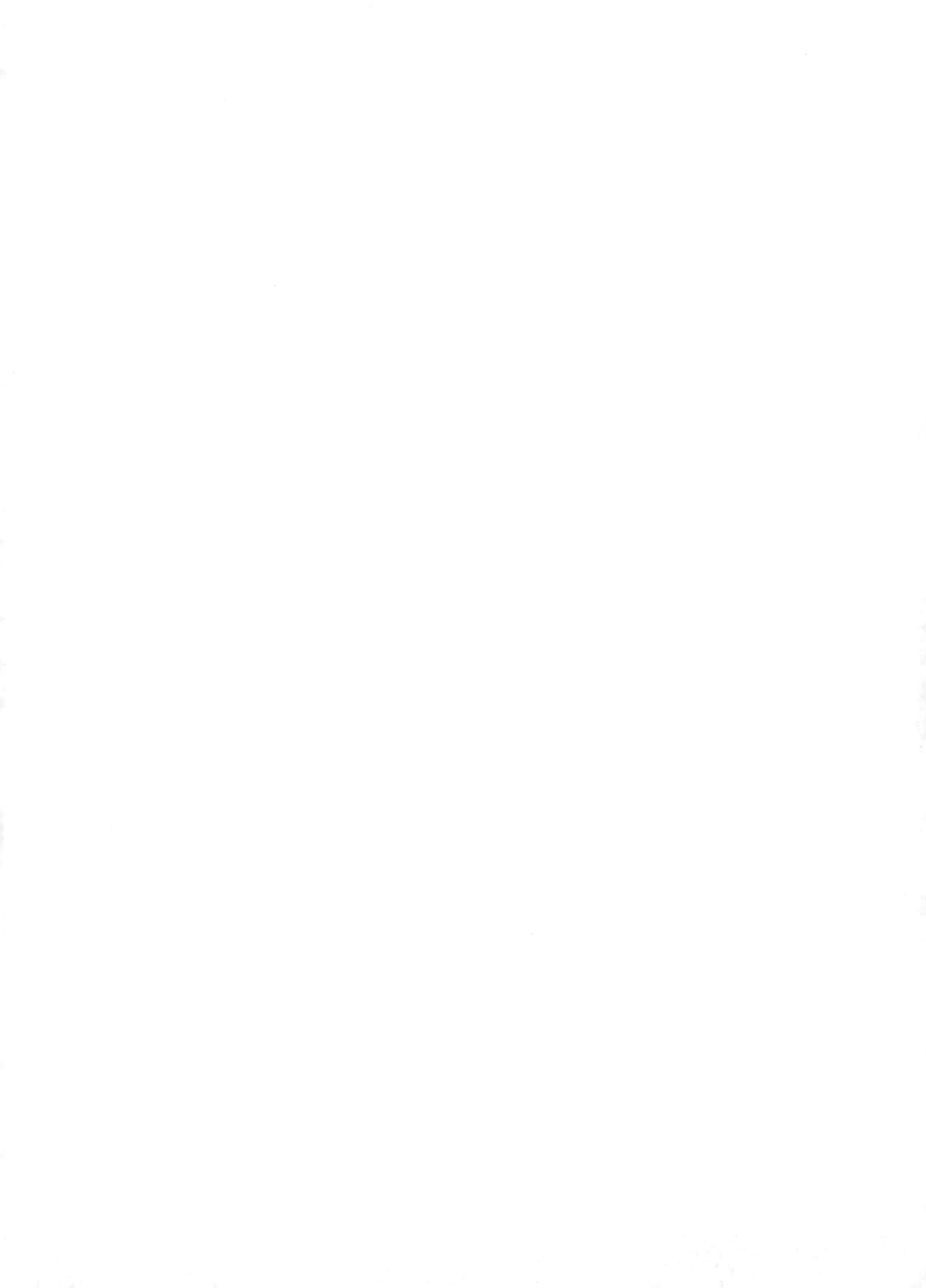